I Can't Stop Shaking

D1073407

More than 10 Million People Suffer with Essential Tremor

By Sandy Kamen Wisniewski

First published by Dog Ear Publishing
4010 W. 86th Street, Ste H
Indianapolis, IN 46268
www.dogearpublishing.net

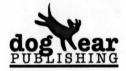

ISBN: 1-59858-091-4
Library of Congress Control Number: 2005936928

This book is printed on acid-free paper.

Printed in the United States of America

For my husband Chuck who loves me tremor and all.

Contents

Foreword

I am proud to recommend this book written by a person who has become not only a very good friend but a worldwide advocate for those with Essential Tremor (ET). Sandy and I first met shortly following the appearance of her article in *Woman's Day* in May of 2001. From that point, I knew Sandy would have a significant impact on positively affecting the lives of those with ET. Sandy has certainly risen to the occasion and continues to make a difference.

I have a great deal of respect and admiration for Sandy. She has begun a long journey—a journey to bring awareness about ET to all parts of the world. She has overcome her reluctance to speak out about ET and, in so doing, works diligently to bring about an understanding and normalcy to people whose lives who are filled with frustration trying to perform daily activities that others without ET often take for granted. Activities such as putting on mascara or eye shadow, shaving, eating, drinking, brushing teeth, and even teeing up a golf ball can produce significant difficulty, humiliation, and embarrassment. Activities such as these hold a special meaning to those with a tremor.

This is a wonderful book filled with the experiences and challenges of those who seek to overcome the disabling affects of ET in a world where there are few medications available and virtually none developed for ET. The book is an excellent resource of medical information and is filled with suggestions for coping from those that have lived with tremor for many years.

If you have ET or a tremor of some type that has yet to be diagnosed, you will more than likely identify with the stories that have so readily been shared. Hopefully, through these stories, you will gain your own strength and the encouragement to find ways to make a difference in your life as well as in the lives of others.

Lastly, there is a special bond that forms among people who share the challenges that a chronic medical condition often brings. I hope you, too, will find that special bond with those that have shared their stories and in so doing will help you find a lifetime of peace and solace within.

Thank you, Sandy, for your perseverance. The world needs more people like you who use their talent to bring about positive change. Congratulations on your book and in giving the world this wonderful gift.

Catherine Rice

Executive Director

International Essential Tremor Foundation

Chapter 1
Medical Information on Essential Tremor

The following is taken from a question and answer session with neurologist Peter A. LeWitt and author Sandy Kamen Wisniewski. Dr. Peter A LeWitt was graduated from Brown University in 1972. He earned a Masters in Medical Science and M.D. from Brown in 1975. His practice, the Clinical Neuroscience Center, is located in Southfield, Mich. He is a neurologist who sub-specializes in movement disorders. Dr. LeWitt has been practicing neurology and been involved with Essential Tremor since 1980. Dr. Peter A. LeWitt can be contacted at:

Clinical Neuroscience Center
26400 W. 12 Mile Rd., Ste. 110
Southfield, MI 48034
(248) 355-3875

Q. What is Essential Tremor?

A. By definition, ET is a characteristic rhythmic shaking of muscles caused by the central nervous system. Typically this occurs during action, as, for example, a hand reaching for an object. The regular rhythmic movements of ET are separate from any other malfunctions of the brain's motor system; hence, the term "essential" (which means tremor and nothing else). ET is initiated by signals from one or more centers in the brain, activating the involved muscle groups which are following instructions to contract in a regular manner, at rates typically between four to five times per second. This results in regular oscillations that, in the hand, are experienced as "shaking" or "jerking." Tremor is not the same thing as in coordination, although the net result might be the same. In fact, tremor can be distinguished from a number of categories of involuntary movement. Commonly, ET can be confused with the tremor often seen in Parkinson's disease (PD). The tremor in PD typically occurs with the limbs at rest, while in ET, the resting component is usually absent and tremor arises only during an action of that limb. Tremor brought out by handwriting is typical of ET but not so in PD.

Most commonly, ET affects one or more upper extremities. It can also affect the neck muscles (resulting in head tremor) or the muscles of the larynx involved in generating speech. Less commonly, tremors in this disorder affect the legs, the chin region, or all locations simultaneously.

ET is a common and clearly recognizable clinical syndrome. It lacks any specific test to prove it (other than recordings that can record its frequency and other physical features, which might help to define the condition in contrast to other neurological disorders resembling it). Neurological testing that picture the brain, such as CAT and MRI scans, or EEG recordings, do not show abnormalities in ET. Blood test results also do not show abnormalities in this condition.

Q. Who is most likely to get ET?
A. ET can arise at any age, but it usually appears after the third decade. The most common age of onset for ET is in the same age range that PD also develops, in the sixth decade of life. There is an increasing incidence of ET with age, and once someone develops this condition, it almost never goes away.

Q. Is ET hereditary?
A. There is strong evidence for a hereditary component to this condition in up to half of cases. Interest from first-order relatives occurs in a manner that suggests ET to be an autosomal dominant disorder in its hereditary manifestations. This means that each offspring (male or female) of a parent with the gene for ET (whether the parent manifests this condition or

not) has a 50 percent chance of also possessing the gene. Having the ET gene (or genes) doesn't necessarily mean someone will experience this disorder, but there are certainly family trees indicating that up to half of close relatives are affected.

Why this condition isn't present from childhood in all instances is not known. It is also unknown whether instances of apparently sporadic (non-hereditary occurrence) of ET could actually be genetic cases that were not recognized (because other family members were not known to manifest this condition).

It is possible that there might be multiple causes for ET. The increasing incidence in an aging population of tremors might suggest that, in some instances, action tremors of the ET type are an aging phenomenon. Since everybody has a very low-amplitude tremor in the same range as that of ET, one thought is that ET is just an exaggeration of a condition that can be called "physiological," or normal, tremor.

Q. Do more men or women get ET?
A. It's the same number because of autosomal inheritance (described above).

Q. What does ET look like compared to let's say, Parkinson's disease?
A. As mentioned earlier, PD typically has a resting component, that is, tremor occurs when the hands are not engaged in action and the tremor usually ceases

once the hand muscles are intentionally activated in a task, such as reaching. In contrast, ET is usually evident only during such a task. PD almost never has a voice tremor, although ET does.

By definition, ET involves tremor and nothing else in the way of neurological deficits. PD usually has other associated features, such as slowed movements, decreased dexterity, and rigidity of limb muscles. Other neurological disorders that manifest action tremor like ET also have associated problems that can be brought out on a neurological examination. Patients concerned about other conditions sometimes associated with tremor, like multiple sclerosis, alcohol-induced tremors, or cerebellar degeneration, usually have other features readily demonstrable on careful evaluation.

Q. What tests are given to diagnose ET?
A. Usually none are needed. Again, neurological scans and blood tests will show no abnormalities. A neurologist will conduct a simple test to observe the person's movements during a task, such as touching one's hand to one's nose.

Q. Does ET progress?
A. The severity of tremor amplitude can increase with time. Also, the body locations of tremor can evolve. Tremor that affects just one arm can eventually affect the other arm, or voice can become affected a few

years later. In general, however, most people affected with ET have a stable disorder that does not progress for some period of time, typically from a few months to several years.

Q. How severe does the tremor get with age?
A. Though most people with ET don't have a severe disorder, tremor amplitude can increase over time to the point of disability. This is not inevitable with age. As mentioned earlier, most people have a stable disorder.

Q. Have there been any studies on ET?
A. Numerous studies have been conducted throughout the years. The broad categories of these include epidemiological studies (who gets this condition, what age of onset, twin studies, how many relatives are involved, are there environmental factors, how does one ethnic group compare to others, etc.), pharmacological studies (what medications might help to control—or to exacerbate—tremor), physiological (what mechanisms or locations in the brain seem to be responsible for tremor, what are the physical properties of tremor and factors that modify it, etc.) and quality-of-life studies (impact of ET on disability, etc.). Other "high-powered" aspects of modern brain research have been targeting tremor conditions like ET for many years, including the search for animal models of the disorder and genetic testing that might identify susceptibility or mechanisms in the brain involved in the

process of causing ET.

Q. What is the typical age that ET becomes noticeable?
A. There appears to be a bimodal age distribution for hereditary forms of ET—onset in the 20s and the 50s.

Q. How debilitating can ET become?
A. Although often described as "benign" ET, the tremor can be quite disabling, depending on what body part is affected. A severely tremorous voice, for example, can greatly interfere with someone's livelihood as well as everyday living. Individuals with shaking of the hands, the most common form of ET, may regard it as a nuisance, a social embarrassment, or a disability that requires compensatory maneuvers. In the worst circumstances—a small minority of cases—hand and head tremors can be severe enough to dominate a person's well-being to the point of major disability.

Q. What medications are currently available?
A. There are five groups of medications currently used to help lessen the severity of ET, including benzodiazepines, beta blockers, and anti-seizure medicines like primidone. (See Chapter 2 for further information on ET treatment and medicine.)

Q. What part(s) of the body react the least to medication in controlling the tremor?
A. In general, oral medications don't work all that well

for head or voice tremor. Injections of botulinum toxin (Botox® Therapeutic), however, can help greatly with tremors in these regions.

Q. Do medications work long term?
A. In general, yes.

Q. What about the medical procedure Deep Brain Stimulation (DBS)? What exactly is it, how risky is it, who should consider it, and what kind of results have you seen?
A. I manage several dozen persons who have had DBS for tremor (and many more who have had it for PD). It involves placing small electrodes in tremor-generating centers of the brain that are connected to a stimulator device that puts small currents of electricity to work to suppress tremors. This is a permanent and safe solution to tremor control that offers benefit to the majority of patients who receive it (probably 80 percent to 95 percent have excellent results, regardless of the level of improvement occurring with oral medications or botulinum toxin). It tends to work best for limb tremors rather than head or voice tremor. DBS does carry risks, such as bleeding into the brain, which could cause stroke or death, but these risks are small. Candidates for DBS are those who fail to achieve adequate control with all available medications and whose disability from the disorder is worth the small, but serious, risks involved in this surgical procedure.

Q. Many ET sufferers have reported that their doctors either didn't know they had ET, weren't able to diagnose it, or, even when diagnosed, didn't offer any information about it. Why do you think that is?

A. ET has a low level of awareness on the part of physicians, who can sometimes regard this condition as "normal aging." Physicians may fail to manifest concern about the impact of this condition on a patient's quality of life and may show "therapeutic nihilism" towards some very well-tolerated and effective remedies that can be used chronically to suppress tremor. In addition, this condition is often confused with PD and therefore inappropriate medications are prescribed that do not work for ET.

Q. What about children with ET? Are there statistics on the number of children with ET and treatment suggestions for them?

A. There have been studies in children, who, fortunately, respond to the same medications as adults.

Q. From your experience how do you think ET affects the sufferer?

A. It can range from a minor affliction—not judged by the patient to be worth taking medication regularly—to a major disability that affects all aspects of daily living.

Q. What would you like to see the medical community do better when it comes to ET?
A. Increase awareness, offer patients the maximum in advice and access to the available medication options, and help patients and their families to accommodate the impact of this chronic disorder.

Q. Are certain types of tremor more prevalent in either sex?
A. No.

Q. Is alcohol always an effective temporary cure?
A. No. Only a fraction of patients respond. In addition, the effects are temporary and sometimes not appropriate for everyday situations of tremor.

Q. Is alcoholism a common problem for ET sufferers?
A. No.

Q. Can trauma cause ET? Are there other conditions that may bring it on, certain diseases or disorders, for example, or does anybody really know for sure?
A. The most common manifestation of ET is on a hereditary basis. Head injury and toxic exposure are rare causes of tremor that are usually accompanied by other neurological impairments.

Q. Do you find that patients become social recluses?

A. Rarely, but tremor is a potentially socially stigmatizing disorder that can lead to social withdrawal.

Q. Does the severity of ET vary with hunger, fatigue, etc.?

A. Stressful situations, including exercise and hunger, can temporarily increase the amplitude of tremor. ET can be like a barometer of the emotions.

Q. Could there be a potential single cure or is ET so varied that many cures may be necessary to cover the various types?

A. A cure for a genetically induced disorder may be a tall order. However, highly effective medications that can suppress tremor already exist, and research is searching for more options.

Q. Do you feel that ET is underreported and therefore understudied?

A. Yes.

Chapter 2
Medical Treatment of Essential Tremor

One of the mysterious things about ET is that several seemingly unrelated classes of medications can lessen shaking. Several prescription drugs are routinely used for ET. While one might not work at all, another might be highly effective. Despite extensive tremor research, various drug treatments useful for ET have become known mostly through chance discoveries rather than from knowledge about what brain mechanisms should be targeted by medications.

Under the best circumstances, regular use of one or more of the available medications can offer good control of ET. Each of these drugs should be explored to help find the best treatment.

For people who don't respond adequately to available drugs, surgery (implanting an electrical stimulator or lesioning the brain's tremor pathways in the thalamus) is an option. While tremors associated with Parkinson's disease or that result from injuries to the brain generally do not respond to medications known to be effective for ET, surgery may help.

Alcohol, which can often lessen tremors that occur during movement, is the oldest remedy known to work for ET. Not every patient experiences this effect, however, and the improvement is generally short-lived. For people whose tremor does respond to alcohol, tremor control usually can come from a small, non-intoxicating amount—about a half glass of wine. An alcoholic drink before a meal can help make it easier for some patients who have hand tremor to use utensils.

Because alcohol is rapidly cleared from the system and is not acceptable for everyday use, it is far from perfect as an ET treatment option. Moreover, some patients experience a rebound increase of tremor several hours after drinking an alcoholic beverage.

How alcohol works against tremor is not well understood. In experimental studies, 1-octanol (a compound chemically related to ethanol) has been reported to be effective against ET. Another alcohol-related compound (a European sedative called methylpentynol) was not. However, 1-octanol is still a research medication and is not available. (See the next section for more information on 1-octanol.)

Drugs Used to Treat ET

Beyond alcohol, there are five groups of prescription medications that can help manage tremor. Each of the drugs was developed for other medical purposes and later discovered to have an anti-tremor effect. Among these are a group of drugs—benzodiazepines—that also serve as mild tranquilizers. Another class of anti-tremor drugs is beta blockers, which are most commonly used for high blood pressure and various heart conditions. Other options for treating tremor are methazolamide (Neptazine®), a medication generally used for controlling glaucoma, and two anti-epilepsy drugs: primidone (Mysoline®) and topiramate (Topamax®). Experience has shown that each can be highly successful at tremor control even when there is a lack of response to other drugs. Sometimes the combination of two or more drugs gives the best results.

Neither age, familial occurrence of ET, nor duration of tremor influences a person's likelihood of responsiveness to any particular medication. While these anti-tremor drugs seem to act in the brain at centers where tremor is generated, the calming effect of tranquilizer medications to lessen stress or anxiety (situations that can temporarily make tremor worse) also can be part of their benefit.

Benzodiazepines

Benzodiazepines useful for tremor control include

drugs such as clonazepam (Klonopin®), lorazepam (Ativan®), and diazepam (Valium®). While these reduce tremor, they can cause drowsiness. These drugs are often well tolerated at effective anti-tremor doses. Clonazepam, the most widely used of this group in treating tremor, is typically used at 0.5 mg three times a day for best results.

Beta Blockers

Beta blockers are the oldest class of prescription drugs known to help against ET. The first of these to be used, propranolol (Inderal®), was recognized in the 1960s to be effective. Other drugs such as nadolol (Corgard®) and metoprolol (Lopressor®) also have been used for tremor. Some drugs classed as beta blockers, however, are not effective.

The optimal anti-tremor dose of propranolol and other effective beta blockers is typically less than amounts needed to treat high blood pressure. Although they can have a variety of side effects, beta blockers are generally well tolerated. The usual effective dose range of propranolol for tremor control is 60–120 mg daily in divided doses or one daily dose in a long-acting preparation.

Primidone

Beyond its use in epilepsy, primidone was found to be useful against ET more than 20 years ago. It's one of the most effective drugs and, in some instances, has provided patients with complete control of tremor. Primidone is most effective at a daily intake much lower than amounts generally needed to control epileptic seizures. Usual effective regimens involve divided doses totaling 150–300 mg per day and the pediatric dose form, a 50-mg tablet. Primidone is gradually converted in the body to phenobarbital (another drug used for seizures), but only the parent compound exerts an anti-tremor effect. Initially, primidone can cause drowsiness, but it tends to be well tolerated after a gradual build-up over several weeks. Up to two-thirds of patients with ET respond well to primidone.

Methazolamide

Like the other drugs, methazolamide was also discovered by chance to be effective for some patients with ET. Although this drug is less likely to have a significant anti-tremor effect than beta blockers or primidone, it is an important treatment option because it rarely causes drowsiness or lowers blood pressure. The effective dose is generally 100–300 mg per day.

Additional drugs

In the hope of finding more effective treatments for ET, researchers have conducted dozens of studies to test other drugs that act on the central nervous system. The search has paid off with a few additional options from the anti-convulsant drug class.

Although its effectiveness hasn't been as clearly established as the drugs discussed previously, topiramate has been shown in a published study to help control tremor. Other drugs for which there have been anecdotal experiences of improvements include zonisamide (Zonegran®), levetiracetam (Keppra®), gabapentin (Neurontin®), and the antidepressant mirtazapine (Remeron®). Apart from topiramate, which has undergone relatively large-scale testing, the other drugs haven't been as thoroughly studied for tremor.

In the absence of knowing what the ideal treatment is for ET, scientists and clinicians often test new medications developed for other neurological applications to see if the medications might also suppress tremor. This approach sometimes leads to new treatments.

Medications for tremor control provide only symptomatic relief; they are not a cure. It's important to consider the option of dose adjustment (both amount and timing) to reach the best level of relief and least amount of side effects. Generic versions of these drugs are as effective as brand name products.

Botulinum toxin

Beyond pills, another medication treatment for controlling voice or head (neck) tremor is botulinum toxin (Botox® Therapeutic). When injected in measured amounts into affected muscles, botulinum toxin can exert an anti-tremor effect that lasts for months. Generally, botulinum toxin has not been useful for limb tremors, although there have been rare examples of marked effectiveness.

NIH Study of 1-octanol [1]

While alcohol appears to be one of the most effective ET "treatments"—as many as 80 percent to 100 percent of patients report positive responses—regular alcohol use has potentially serious medical, social, and legal consequences. A special type of alcohol, however, has been shown to improve tremor in animal studies.

The substance, 1-octanol, reduces the rhythmic activity of brain-stem nerve cells thought to cause tremor in ET, and at doses much lower than alcohol. That's good news for two reasons:

1. Not only might 1-octanol be an effective ET treatment, but it also has a lower potential for causing intoxication than does alcohol at an effective dose.

2. 1-octanol may be an alternative to drugs like propranolol and mysoline, whose side effects and effectiveness are often unsatisfactory.

Found naturally in low concentrations in citrus peel, 1-octanol has Food and Drug Administration (FDA) approval for use as a food additive (flavoring agent). It has been used safely for this purpose for many years.

Two National Institutes of Health (NIH) studies using 1-octanol in ET patients show promising results. The first study was done with very low doses of 1-octanol. The second study found an effective dose with no significant side effects.

A third study currently under way uses a double-blind, placebo-controlled approach to further test 1-octanol's effectiveness at doses previously shown to be safe in ET. Study participants all have alcohol-responsive essential tremor.

Conducted at the NIH Clinical Center, this latest study uses a cross-over design, which means patients take both 1-octanol and placebo but in a different order. The study involves two one-week treatment phases with a one-week break between. One group of patients receives 1-octanol in the first treatment phase and placebo in the second, while the other group receives placebo in the first treatment phase and 1-octanol in the second. Patients go home after the first treatment phase and return after one week for the second phase.

An accelerometer mounted on cardboard and taped to the patient's hand measures tremor amplitude.

The study is expected to show significantly reduced tremor in patients who receive 1-octanol as compared to placebo and at a dose that patients should tolerate well.

Deep Brain Stimulation Therapy

For those with a severe tremor who do not respond well to medications, there is a surgical option. Activa® Tremor Control Therapy is delivered by an implanted medical device, similar to a cardiac pacemaker, that uses electrical stimulation to block the brain signals that cause tremor in an upper extremity.

The Activa Tremor Control System stimulates targeted cells in the thalamus—the brain's message relay center—via electrodes that are surgically implanted in the brain and connected to a neurostimulator implanted near the collarbone. The electrical stimulation can be non-invasively adjusted to maximize the therapy's benefit for each patient.

Generally, this therapy is not for the newly diagnosed or those who are doing well on medication. Patients with cognitive problems such as hallucinations, confusion, or memory loss also are not good candidates. Only a doctor experienced with Activa® Therapy can determine whether a person is a good candidate.

Even if your doctor determines you are a candidate, only you and your loved ones can make the final decision to go ahead with the surgery. Research as much information as you can. Try to speak with patients who have Activa Therapy. Make sure you are comfortable with the surgeon who will perform the procedure. Make sure all of your questions are answered. Then carefully weigh the risks and benefits.

The Procedure

Patients who have the Activa System usually describe the surgical procedure as demanding and exhausting, but not painful.

Your surgeon should explain the implant procedure thoroughly so you know what to expect before entering the hospital.

The duration of the procedure and the specific steps involved can vary. The surgery typically lasts four to eight hours beginning with the placement of the stereotactic headframe designed to keep your head stationary and help guide the surgeon in the placement of the lead. Next, the doctor will take an image of your brain using sophisticated imaging equipment like a computed tomography (CT) or magnetic resonance imaging (MRI).

Next you will be given a sedative and a local anesthetic in preparation for the implantation of the lead. It is necessary for you to be awake during this part of the procedure so that you can communicate with your doctor. Fortunately, the brain itself has no pain receptors in it, so you should feel no pain in this area.

Your surgeon will take time to make sure the lead is precisely placed in the area of the brain that will give you the best symptom relief. The surgeon will use a test stimulator to ensure the stimulation relieves symptoms. Depending on your situation, the neurosurgeon may continue by implanting the neurostimulator and extension while you're under general anesthesia. Alternatively, the neurostimulator and extension may be implanted a few days later.

The hospital stay is usually one or two days. Your doctor may wait a few days or weeks to turn on the stimulation.

Chapter 3
I Have Essential Tremor

The following pages are stories of people who live with Essential Tremor. It is in their words, from their hearts, spoken openly and honestly.—Sandy

Detours in Life

By Sandy Kamen Wisniewski

My hands always shook. The tremor became more obvious during my teens. My family and I never really talked about it. I was adopted, so without anyone else shaking in the family, it seemed to me the attitude was just that's the way Sandy is.

During school my tremor embarrassed me in front of my peers, so I learned to hide my hands up my long sleeves or in my pockets. I made a point not to eat at friends' homes or if I did, I ate only food that could be held easily. In school I learned to slide papers over surfaces when I needed to pass them on—handing them to someone would have made the tremor more noticeable.

I was a shy, introverted girl with a few close friends. Having a tremor and being shy only made me more insecure. With my close friends, though, I felt at ease and hid my tremor far less.

I wrote in block letters, script was too difficult. The loops on the script would look shaky and, to me, very ugly. I learned to press the pen hard on the paper to make writing easier. Most of the tricks I learned early in my life I continued using as I grew up.

When I was 14, my tremor got much worse. When I was upset, which was often (I was a teenager after all), my tremor would rev up, causing me terrible embarrassment if I was with people. I was sure it was psychological. My self-esteem at that time in my life was low to begin with, so I often thought to myself, "What an idiot I am, I can't even control myself from shaking." I didn't know what I had and because my family was so nonchalant about it I thought, "Well it must not be a big deal then." But I have learned since then, it IS a big deal. And it took me almost 20 years to figure that out.

At the same time my tremor was getting worse, I was pestering my parents about looking for my birth mother. My parents were always open to the idea of finding my biological mother but wanted to wait until I was older. However with the tremor getting worse, they felt strongly it was time to find my birth mother—if for no other reason than to find out about my genetic health history.

My parents found my birth mother when I was 14 and we asked her about the tremor. She said that no one in her family shook, so concerned, my parents sent me to a neurologist. After some simple tests, such as holding my arms out in front of me palms down, and then with my arms outstretched, touching my fingers to my nose, the doctor diagnosed me with Essential Tremor. I left the office knowing what I had, but with the impression that once again, it was no big deal. I was never given any information about it nor did he explain the long-term effects of it. So I continued to assume I was the only one who had it and because the doctor didn't seem to be concerned at all, once again it was no big deal.

In my mid-teens, I started working in restaurants and bars. At first I was a waitress but carried mostly pizzas and heavy plates to the table, which was easy to do. I became close friends with the restaurant manager, so when glasses filled with drinks or coffee with saucers had to be handled, she was kind enough to do it for me. It was a very small restaurant and we were the only two people working there, so it was easy and fun.

After that restaurant closed, I worked at a series of restaurants and bars as a cocktail waitress. I learned to hold the glasses in a way that made it possible to deliver them without spilling. My main objective was not to get stressed out, which would make the tremor worse.

One day I was running late for work. I had found that is the WORST possible thing for my tremor. I hurried inside, punched in, and got right to work. My internal tremor—the tremor I feel inside but no one sees—was distracting and in overdrive. I looked at my hands and saw the trembling. "Oh, no," I thought, a lump growing in my throat. "How am I going to pull this off?" I took a deep breath and headed for a table with three men and three women in their late 20s. I greeted them, smiled, and asked them what I could get for them. Aware that I was unable to write the drink order on a pad, I relied on my memory to get the order right.

The bartender prepared the six margaritas (a bad choice for my trembling hands). I put them on a tray and, carefully holding the tray, I headed for the table. Knowing full well I was not going to be able to hold the tray with one hand while I picked up the drinks and put each one on the table with the other, I opted to put the whole tray and drinks on the table in front of them and slide each drink off the tray and in front of each person. It looked like an unorthodox way to provide service, but I figured that at least I wouldn't spill.

They intently watched my hands shaking. My face was burning with embarrassment. After all the drinks were served, one of the men looked at my hands and then scanned me slowly from head to toe. With a smirk on his face, he said, "Honey, do we make you nervous?" The whole group erupted in laughter. I rushed away from the table, my eyes stinging with tears.

By the far side of the bar, I was seething. My chest felt heavy with anger. "How dare them!" I said between clenched teeth. Without another moment of thought, I strode purposely towards their table.

Their social chatter stopped. With all their attention on me, I leaned far over the table. My face expressionless, I said in a low voice, "You want to know why I am shaking? Because I have only six months to live." With great dramatic flare I hung my head, sighed, and walked away. Looking back over my shoulder and seeing their stunned faces I thought, "That taught them."

When I was 19, I started my first business, an in-home pet sitting service I called, The Pet Sitters of America. During the first year, I juggled the business and two or three part-time restaurant jobs. After quitting a cocktail waitress job, I heard that a restaurant located down the block was looking for waitresses. Everyone told me the money was good so I applied.

The first day at work I learned that the wait staff was required to carry plates up and down their arms (they didn't allow trays). Coffee cups and soup bowls with saucers were very popular staples at that restaurant. My first night I struggled to and from the kitchen to the dining area, my arm and hand loaded with various plates, bowls, and cups. My hands and arms were shaking so badly that the clanking, clattering, and spills stopped all conversations in the entire restaurant each time I entered the room. Customers were grabbing food items from me as quickly as they could, trying to avoid getting hot soup, coffee, or whatever spilled all over their business-casual dress. Some would hastily move their chairs back from the table as I refilled coffee cups. One man took my hand and said, with great sincerity, "Sweetie, relax." The next day I walked in preparing to quit, but the owner beat me to it. He slipped me a 20 and said, "Now you take care."

By then my business was growing to the point that I didn't need to work as many other jobs, so I concentrated on building my business and worked just one additional job.

In 1989, when I was 22, I married my boyfriend Chuck and began working Pet Sitters full time. In a short time I had my first child, Sarah. When she was a newborn, it took my clumsy hands time to get used to the small motor skills necessary to take care of my baby. Dressing her in her tiny clothes was very difficult and time consuming. But luckily for me I did all my chores of caring for her—clothing, diapering, feeding, bathing—when no one else was around, so I didn't have to suffer the terrible embarrassment of my shaky hands.

My son Danny was born 17 months after Sarah and I was extremely busy taking care of my kids and running a new business. Chuck worked full time so everything else fell on me. In 1993 the business had grown so large that Chuck quit his job and went into business with me. By that time I was feeling unfulfilled, burned out, and in need of a change.

That same year I decided that I was going to go back to college, study acting, and become an actress—my lifelong dream and passion. I envisioned starting with commercials and working my way up to major television shows. By this time I had also been doing more and more freelance writing (I have to type with two fingers, hunt-and-peck style) and had gotten some articles published. I even saw myself writing and starring in plays or television sitcoms. My attitude was, "It is never too late to start anew!"

Pumped up and ready to go, I arrived at my first acting class. With the class sitting in a circle on the floor, our teacher explained that she wanted us to get comfortable improvising by doing some improvisation games. She told the men, "I want you to pretend you are shaving. I want you to show different emotions while you do it, such as being happy, sad, anxious, scared, etc. Ladies, I want you to pretend to apply makeup. Also, show different emotions."

I watched one-by-one my classmates play-acting. When it came to my turn, I lifted my hands to my face. As I pretended to put on my makeup, my hands looked like they were jolting uncontrollably. As strange as it sounds, I didn't even think that my tremor would make this exercise impossible. For all those years I had learned to hide my tremor. I hadn't had many public situations arise in the past six years to cause me to see my tremor as a handicap or embarrassment so I guess I just forgot. But there it was in full view of a room full of strangers. The girl with no control, with horribly, deformed hands for the entire world to see—at least that's how I felt. After just a few seconds (which felt like an eternity), I dropped my hands and clasped them together in my lap. The students looked at me puzzled by what had just happened. After the last student finished, I excused myself and left the classroom.

I went straight to my car, sunk low in the seat, and sobbed. I came to realize that day that for years I had hidden my tremor the same way I had when I was a kid. I avoided social situations and when I couldn't, I made excuses not to eat or drink and left early. Part of me was confused by my reaction. I imagine that other people would look at me sitting in my car so upset and say, "So what? What's the big deal anyway?" But now I knew I wouldn't be able to be an actress. There was no way. Actresses have to carry things and use their hands all the time. There was no way I could hide the shaking on film or stage.

Arriving home, I called my birth mother to spill my guts. She was the only person I felt I could talk to without judgment. I told her what had happened and she said, "I'm crying with you, Sandy. If I could take it away, I would. If I could have it instead of you, I would." We went on to talk about the mystery of how I got ET. She said she was sure my birth father never shook. She also reflected on her childhood and her parents and once again said that she didn't recall anyone shaking on her side either.

I decided I didn't want to give up on my dream of acting after all. Shortly thereafter I got a prescription for Inderol from my doctor and I began taking it in the hopes my tremor would disappear. Then I could resume my acting career. My doctor told me to gradually increase the dose until I no longer shook. After a week, my tremor disappeared, which was an awesome feeling. However within days, I developed a terrible side effect: Severe leg cramps made me unable to walk for days. My doctor said cramps were not a typical side effect of the medication I was taking. I stopped the medication. The cramps went away. The tremor came back.

After a week of feeling sorry for myself, I did what was typical for me—I did not give up. I decided I was going to find a way to act anyway. I saw a newspaper ad looking for people interested in learning to be a professional clown. I thought it would be a perfect way to get involved in acting. I reasoned that I would be less nervous because I would be wearing a mask. Besides, what small motor skills were involved in clowning anyway? I started clown school the next week.

What I learned from my time at clown school was that practically everything you do in clowning requires small motor skills. Applying makeup was tedious and detailed. I would place my elbows on a table, grab my right wrist with my left hand and slowly, very slowly, draw the fine lines around my mouth and eyes. Over time I became proficient, but I allowed myself twice the amount of time my classmates needed to apply the face. I learned face painting, balloon sculpturing, and simple magic tricks. I named my character Sunshine and perfected her outfit and unique facial makeup.

My first clown job was two hours of balloon sculpturing at a local forest preserve for a company party. It was hot and humid and about 15 kids were waiting impatiently in line from the get-go. Because I felt pressured to hurry and it was hot, my tremor was really bad. To top that off, the balloons began breaking one after the other (I found out later it was due to the heat). It was a complete disaster. By the time I left, the kids were looking at me like I was some shaking, freaky clown from another planet. Those kids who were already borderline scared of clowns could now confirm that they had a reason to be scared. I realized I could no longer do balloon sculpturing—I cared too much about kids to traumatize any more of them.

My next assignment was to do face painting at a

summer community party. What I drew looked like a globby mess, but the children and their parents were kind enough to thank me before hurrying away. Pretty soon I was sitting at the picnic table alone—obviously the other parents had seen or heard of my handwork and wisely avoided me. I was terribly embarrassed and discouraged. I'm sure they thought I was a clown on drugs.

I did discover a few things I could do as a clown. I could walk in parades and make people laugh at my silly antics and I could lead party games such as duck, duck, goose; hot potato; and tag. I was a funny, sweet, innocent, silly clown with a high, crackly voice. I loved being Sunshine the Clown and entertaining crowds. After a year and a half of clowning, I decided to stop. I'm proud to say I stopped not because of my tremor (although maybe that should have been why for all those kids' sakes!), but simply because I wanted to move on to other things.

During the time I was clowning, my birth mother Lil started experiencing what she thought was her heart beating too fast and, as she put it, "some sort of weird internal feeling." It scared her enough to see a doctor. Her husband Lee also had noticed that her head shook when she was concentrating on something like reading or writing. Her doctor diagnosed her with Essential Tremor. When we spoke on the phone, she said that the internal shaking was distracting and a bit scary. I told her, "Welcome to the world of Essential

Tremor." Then I assured her she would get used to the feeling. Since that time her head tremor has worsened and a tremor has started in her hands.

One day while at Pet Sitter's office, my assistant Darcy handed me a tiny newspaper clipping that she had saved for me from a local paper. It read:

> *The Essential Tremor Support Group in Skokie will be having a guest speaker—a neurologist who will be providing information about Essential Tremor.*

I was floored. I looked at Darcy and said, "I can't believe they have a support group. I thought I was the only one who has this!" I wasn't alone!

I arrived for the meeting in a small auditorium at the Skokie Public Library. I watched as people signed in. Some people couldn't because of ET and had someone do it for them. Most of the people there were at least 30 years older than me and had very visible hand, head, and voice tremors. I took a seat all the way in the back of the room and listened intently to the doctor as she went through her presentation.

Never having known anything other than a name for my condition, I learned a lot about the disorder that had plagued me since childhood. I couldn't believe more than 10 million people have Essential Tremor! Where were they? Why didn't I know any of them? I also observed that day a lot of gray and white heads in front of me bobbing up and down and side to side. The idea that I too would someday be that disabled scared me terribly so I decided to write about it.

When I got home, for the first time ever, I wrote about my life living with Essential Tremor. The next week I presented the story to my writers' support group for their input. As I read my story out loud I was nervous and embarrassed, but anxious to hear what my peers thought of my story. When I finished, everyone said they were very surprised that I shook. I told them that it was years and years of practice hiding it. One of the participants, who had written for many medical publications suggested that I try to get it published. She said she believed it would sell because it was an unusual topic.

I took her advice and sent it off to four major magazines. Within a month I got an e-mail from an editor from *Woman's Day* magazine. They wanted the story! During my research for the story, I learned about the International Essential Tremor Foundation (IETF) and spoke to their Executive Director, Cathy Rice, numerous times. We formed an immediate bond. When the story hit the newsstands, initially I felt exposed and vulnerable. But I knew that the story had to be told, that people needed to know they weren't alone. The response I received was very positive and accepting. I began getting letters from people around the country that suffered with ET. Some of them hid it, like I had. Others said they lived in isolation and thought that they were the only one. I was so deeply touched by their heart-felt letters that I decided to help the IETF by spreading the word about ET. I wrote an article for one of our local weekly newspapers by The Pioneer Press and was featured in the local daily newspaper, *The News-Sun*. I also began speaking to many business and civic groups.

Whenever I began my speech I started by asking, "Does anyone know why Kathryn Hepburn shakes?" Invariably I heard, "Parkinson's disease." "No," I would say, "She had what's called Essential Tremor. Who here has heard of Essential Tremor, raise your hand?" Each and every time, no one raised his or her hand.

One of my speaking engagements was especially important for me. I was given five minutes before a keynote speaker at my home chamber of commerce. I had just stepped down from the presidency of the chamber and was ready to reveal to everyone that I had ET.

After being introduced by the chamber's current president, I walked up to the front of the room and began as I always did. As I expected, no one raised his or her hand. After completing my speech I sat in my seat, relieved that it was over; I no longer had to keep my secret. I went back to my chair flooded with relief.

Illinois State Senator Terry Link, the keynote speaker, made his way to the podium and began, "Sandy, you asked if anyone knew what Essential

Tremor is." I thought, "Why is he saying that to me?" He went on, "I know exactly what Essential Tremor is because I have it also." He went on to talk about how he too had hidden it from everyone except his family and some key people who work for him. He said as a kid, classmates called him "Shaky" and as an adult, he had been accused of being an alcoholic.

I sat there stunned, a lump growing in my throat. This was very strange. This must be one more way that someone up above is telling me to keep speaking up about ET, I thought. Afterwards, Senator Link offered me his card and said, "Call me if I can do anything at all." I took him up on his offer and he was kind enough to join me for some public speaking engagements. We also had a full-page article in *The News-Sun* that talked about our struggles with ET and educated the reader about what ET was and where to go to get additional information. Senator Link has been a wonderful advocate for our cause of getting the word out about ET ever since and I venture to guess that he has also personally grown from the experience.

Nowadays, I choose to consider myself blessed—tremor and all. Because of Essential Tremor, I experienced performing as a clown, having an article published in a major magazine (which in the writing world is a huge accomplishment), and meeting some wonderful people along the way. As far as acting goes, it wasn't in the cards. Now that I'm older and wiser I think I wouldn't have loved it that much anyway. Having ET is a hardship, I admit, but rather than dwell on the negatives, I choose to see it as a challenge. And I love challenges.

Finally, I thought I'd share some of the ways I have learned to compensate for my limitations:

- I never measure ingredients in recipes with small measuring spoons. I have gotten good at guessing and just shaking a bit of this or that in the batter.

- I ask someone else to paint my nails.

- I ask people to help me with things I can't do myself.

- I allow extra time to apply makeup.

- I eat soup with a big, heavy spoon.

- I drink my coffee from a big, heavy mug.

- When I speak publicly, if something has to be written on a board, I write it beforehand. If that isn't possible, I ask for a volunteer to write, joking that the board "doesn't have spell check" or that "my handwriting would defeat the purpose of writing on the board to begin with 'cause no one will be able to read it."

- I try to remain calm because getting upset makes my tremor much worse. (I think that would be a good principle even if I didn't have ET!)

- I send my family to a hairdresser instead of cutting their hair myself. I nicked my husband's ear one too many times!

- It's impossible for me to type the traditional way; instead I have learned to be a very fast two-finger typist.

- I program my mouse so that it's not so sensitive to movement.

- I plan ahead if I am going to a social event. If I have to go without someone to help me, I eat before I go in case I can't hold a plate. Then when I get there, if wine is available, I have a glass so my tremor is calmed and I can enjoy the next few hours. If my husband, Chuck, is with me, he carries the plate for me.

Leave The Peas Please

By James C. Lambert

Throughout the early part of my life I vaguely realized that there was something wrong with my manual dexterity. I could never color within the lines in coloring books, which would lower my grades. In high school, much to my chagrin, I made one C. (That C kept me from being the Salutatorian of my class, by the way.) The embarrassing C was earned in typing class. I was a fast typist, but I had trouble hitting the correct keys;

wrong keys meant lower grades. In the 1950s, the mistakes were all recorded right on that white page with no way to erase or hide them. If I concentrated and tried to type very slowly and deliberately, I could minimize the mistakes.

The other significant thing I learned was that I was not going to be an athlete. Football and especially basketball were not my forte. I participated in these activities with shaking hands, but I never realized that the errant passes, missed shots, and poor coordination may have been related to the shaking. I realized that this problem seemed to be almost uniquely my own — none of my friends had it. I decided that I must be nervous. It was an easy diagnosis to make, because my mother and her brother both suffered from "nervous problems," a euphemism for mental illness at the time. Even though my uncle and my mother had these terrible "nervous problems," *their* hands didn't shake. My nervous problem, I surmised, was manifesting in a different way.

In college, I began drinking coffee but my right hand could not hold a cup steady enough to prevent the appearance of brown dribbles on my shirt. Since spilling coffee in social situations was a continual embarrassment, I stopped drinking coffee. In the 50s and 60s, you were considered a little different if you didn't drink coffee, but I felt that being considered different was preferable to the embarrassment of spills.

After college I was drafted into the United States

Army. Even though I had been trained to use hunting rifles while growing up, I was a terrible marksman during Army training — I could not hold the long rifle steady enough to aim properly. To supplement my meager Army pay, I took a part-time job as a bar waiter. It lasted two evenings. I could not hold the glasses without shaking and, to avoid spilling drinks, I served the drinks very slowly. I quit before they fired me.

At around 40, my shaking, which had worsened, forced me to learn to eat with my left hand. Fatigue and hunger dramatically intensified the shaking. At around the same time my left hand began to join the ranks of the nervous. I was concerned I was developing serious health problems.

In my early 50s, I noticed that my shaking was very bad in the middle of the day when I was hungry. I began to avoid having lunch with anyone. If it wasn't possible to avoid lunch, my menu choices had nothing to do with what appealed to me. They were choices dictated by what food I could eat without spilling or dropping. At dinnertime, however, I never had a problem with the shaking. This made no sense and was a nagging mystery.

There have been other interesting things that are difficult for me to do. Common ones include:

Brushing my teeth

Clipping my finger nails

Shaving (If I had a heavy beard, I might need occasional blood transfusions.)

Putting keys in locks

Taking one page of paper from a stack or turning the thin pages of a dictionary

Using the tiny keyboard of cell phones and other small electronic devices

Using an ATM where the touch screen commands are small (for example, missing the withdrawal button and hitting deposit)

Using a mouse or any other device that requires precise movement

Coping with these inconveniences is a learning experience. For example, I hold the mouse with both hands when I am having difficulty. It may look funny to see someone moving such a small device with two hands, but that is what I have to do.

At 54, and with growing concern that I might have Parkinson's disease, I sought medical help. I wanted to know why my shaking was worsening. After an exam by my doctor he scheduled me to see a neurologist. He assured me that the shaking was not Parkinson's disease because of the nature of my tremor, but he wanted a neurologist to verify what I did have.

The neurologist also solved the mystery of my shake-free dinners. He asked if I had alcohol with or before dinner. I told him I nearly always drink a beer or two before dinner. He explained that alcohol calms my tremor. One beer is good for an almost steady hand for thirty minutes or so, although as time has passed and the tremor has grown worse, alcohol has become less effective.

The neurologist thought I was an interesting case because I exhibit certain characteristics that he referred to as "Parkinsonisms." I curl my right arm across my abdomen as though I am hugging myself, like a Parkinson's patient might, when I fear losing my balance. And, like Parkinson's patients, I have severe balance problems. Seeing the look of dread on my face, he assured me that having Parkinsonisms didn't mean that I have Parkinson's disease.

My balance problems are a family legend. At the age of 40 and in excellent health, I completely remodeled the house we lived in. But while replacing the roof on this huge abode, I fell off three times. I must have a guardian angel, because I fell into a lush hedge twice and caught a ladder to break my fall the other time. Recently, my wife has banned me from any unguardrailed heights and I have to get special permission to ascend a ladder.

I have fallen many times for no apparent reason, especially while jogging. I once fell in front of a woman who was walking her dog. She was the most surprised-looking person I have ever seen. She witnessed a man jogging along one minute and then falling the next for no apparent reason. Many people have seen me fall. I firmly believe that they thought I was drunk.

An interesting thing about my tremor is that I can be sitting, perhaps reading, and experience no noticeable tremor whatsoever. Any change in my environment — as insignificant as the noiseless arrival of one of my cats — will start the tremor.

Before my tremor was noticeable to anyone but me, I had a "tap the fender" accident one day. Although there was no visible damage, the other driver insisted that we exchange names and addresses in case some mechanical difficulty surfaced later. This was the first occasion where I was unable to write my name and address. The man must have thought it was strange that I could not write my name and address. He refused to write it down for me. I eventually was able, by placing paper on the hood of his car and holding the pen with both hands.

I began wearing a medical bracelet a few years ago. It identifies me as having essential tremor and lists my address and phone number. I have two specific reasons for wearing the bracelet. I am afraid that people will think that I am drunk and also I need an explanation in case I can't sign my name.

The medical bracelet has an unexpected bonus. A year or so ago, I attended a fancy wedding reception and in the stand-up phase I went to the bar to get a beer. I requested the beer to be served in a bottle. The bartender told me that bottles were against the rules. My explanation of a possible spill did not convince her. So I produced the medical bracelet and told her I had a neurological condition and that I was protected by the Americans with Disabilities Act. She capitulated and I got my beer in the bottle.

This major victory was soon overshadowed by the harsh realities of eating dinner. Pouring the salad dressing from the little salad dressing pitchers used at those events, buttering a roll while sitting elbow-to-elbow with strangers, baring a baked potato that has been wrapped tightly in aluminum foil, are all challenges at a formal dinner. With the help of my wife and the use of my left hand, I was able to complete dinner with no major embarrassments, and with the peas left on the plate.

Essential Tremor has affected me in unexpected ways. For example, I could not function as a communion minister at my church. I realized when I went to the training session that I would not be able to handle the tiny wafers and could not hold a full cup of wine without spilling some of it. After initial disappointment, I was relieved that I didn't continue the service training because I would have embarrassed myself with my shaking hands in front of lots of people.

Essential Tremor has changed my life's work. I

had never planned to retire from my career in commercial real estate. But my tremor became very noticeable and I assume that the people I encounter will see the tremor and think that I have suffered physical and perhaps mental deterioration. My lip tremors sometimes, but when it does I cannot feel it. Every time I talk to a stranger I wonder if they are listening to what I am saying or merely watching my lip quivering.

So, I have decided to make my living as a writer. I work in the privacy of my home office and I can use a device (my computer) that can automatically correct my mistakes. Not only does it automatically correct many typos, but it also has a wonderful tool called the "undo" button. I sometimes make major errors that can be undone by the undo. Writing allows me to be insulated from constant contact with the general public and the many situations that cause my tremor to worsen. I will no longer have to stand in front of a group of people and attempt to get a key into a lock, nor fumble with information packets. I will never allow Essential Tremor to defeat me, but it will obviously continue to change my life as it continues to worsen over time.

I happen to be blessed with a very understanding and helpful family. My wife is quick to step in anytime she feels that I will have difficulty serving myself or performing some intricate task.

After my diagnosis, I went through a phase where

I felt I should mention in casual conversations the fact that I have a tremor. I thought it would help people to understand the condition better plus inform the general public. I soon learned that people don't want to hear about my tremor, they want to talk about their own health problems (some of which are laughable compared to genuine health problems). So I don't talk about my tremor unless I am asked about it, or if I need to explain why I can't do certain things. I firmly believe that I have a neurological disorder and not a condition that I should be ashamed of or embarrassed about. When I drop something, or stumble at an inappropriate time, I usually make a humorous remark like, "Hire the handicapped. They're fun to watch."

Since I love beer I decided that I would use it as a temporary cure only in rare situations when a steady hand is required. I will drink a beer to calm my tremor before a social occasion only if it is an event where alcohol is served and if I am already at the event. On weekends I drink a beer if I am going to perform an intricate task such as installing electrical outlets. (My hobby of doing electrical work is almost over.) However, over time the effectiveness of the alcohol continues to decline.

I consider myself fortunate that I can make a living where shaky hands and balance problems are minimal inconveniences and not career-threatening. This is not the case with many professions. I do my best to enjoy my life because even with the tremor I am much better off health-wise than millions of others.

Essential Tremor is not all that bad when you consider what some people have to deal with. Cancer, arthritis, paralysis, and countless other maladies, diseases, and conditions are much worse. I have learned a lot from relatives who have suffered from some terrible physical conditions. None of them complain, so I won't either.

"Shaky" Fox

By Duane Fox

I have lived with Essential Tremor since I was 16 years old. It took me 30 years to discover why I shook. Tremor first appeared in my hands in high school while shooting basketball and later playing golf. Soon writing and eating became increasingly difficult. While attending college I developed a slight head tremor. I discovered early in my college days that a couple of beers seemed to relieve my tremor. Wow, what a benefit. It was amazing how the tremor would disappear: A couple of drinks before class or dinner and no tremor.

My career path was in the music and broadcast industry. Entertaining advertising clients and record executives kept me in the fast lane for more than 20 years. My friends and family just thought I was the nervous type, shaking here and there along the way. As time passed, the shaking seemed to increase. Writing and eating became more difficult. Some days I couldn't sign my name or hold a fork. Eating out became an embarrassment, and shaving in the morning was always an adventure. Electric razors replaced disposable ones; fast-food drive-through windows kept me away from sit-down restaurants.

I remember playing golf with a client one morning. I shook so bad I couldn't tee up my golf ball. A quick stop in the 19th hole and a couple of beers later—bingo! I'm cured. Well, I think you know where my story is heading. After 20 years of drinking to control my tremor, I developed a dependency on alcohol. No amount of alcohol could control my tremor. My alcohol abuse almost killed me.

I had never heard of Essential Tremor, or "ET" as it is called. My doctor first diagnosed me with depression and prescribed antidepressants. I was a 43-year-old, overweight, two-pack-a-day smoker who shook like a leaf. My diet consisted of cigarettes, coffee, alcohol, and fast food. My health and life seemed to be headed downhill. I landed in a treatment center for alcohol abuse. My name there was "Shaky."

But this story doesn't end tragically; it has one of those happy endings filled with hope. I found a doctor who changed my life, one who made me take responsibility for my condition and deal with it. He said there was no cure for my tremor, but if I took certain steps—life-changing ones—I could manage my condition and live and enjoy a normal life.

I no longer smoke or drink caffeine, and I am on a strict diet with little, if any, sugar. Alcohol is a no-no for me, and I exercise daily. My shaking is not an embarrassment for me anymore; I accept that I have a disease and manage it the best I can. My tremor is controlled and helped by my lifestyle and some medication. I play golf, eat out with my family, and enjoy life. If I get shaky, well that's OK today.

I thought I shook all those years because I drank; instead, I drank because I shook. My hope is that others will seek help for their condition, and that the medical profession will continue its research into Essential Tremor. For all of us who never knew why or what made us shake, there is hope. It starts with you and me.

I Hate It!

By Anonymous

I am 51 years old and I have ET. I hate it!!! Years ago before I knew I had it, I noticed my mom's head shaking all the time. I asked her why her head shook. She said, "Oh, I had an auto accident years ago."

When my head starting shaking in my 30s, I said something isn't right here. So I saw a neurologist who diagnosed me with ET. That was when I realized my mom had it, too. It's hereditary.

Now at age 52, I have dystonia along with the ET. My mom has vocal spasmodic dystonia. I have cervical dystonia, which pulls my neck (along with the tremor) to the right. It's so painful!

I recently went for Botox injections and that did not help at all. I wish they would find a cure for this. I hate it. Not only am I embarrassed by it, but I also fear what the rest of my life will be like and how much worse it will get.

Why Am I Different?

By Jan Bolick

Through a Child's Eyes

I am so excited. Being an only child didn't give me a lot of friends, except the ones at church. I am seven years old and this is my first day at school. Boy, look at all these kids and all this stuff! Mom is filling out a bunch of papers—all the mothers are. We are supposed to look around and play with each other. I start playing with another group of girls and it is so much fun. They talk and play rather than sit and do nothing like my dolls. I am having so much fun and we are going to have snacks and drinks. I already know I'm going to love school. I am one of the big kids now.

Hey, cookies with sprinkles and orange drink—WOW!

We all get in line and there is this girl and her name is the same as mine. That's great—we can be sisters. It's my turn. This lady gives me a little paper plate with two cookies and tells me to get a cup of orange drink from the next lady. I have my cookies in one hand and reach out to take my drink. Oops—my hand shakes some and the drink gets on my cookies. This lady is a grouch and she tells me to eat them anyway. That's OK, they're just a little wet.

I am very careful walking to the table so I won't get any of my drink on the floor. OH NO! Now my other hand shakes a little and the paper plate lets a cookie fall off. It's the dry one. I'm at the table and sit down beside Jan. I take a bite of my cookie. Not so good with orange drink on it, but Mom said to use my best manners so I'll eat it anyway. I want to taste my drink so I take a drink. One of the other girls asks me why I'm still a baby. "You hold your cup with both hands like my little brother. Baby Janice." I told her I didn't want to spill anymore. She laughs at me and tells me to "Get a bottle—baby." OK, I don't like her. She has ugly hair. Nobody else says anything mean but they stare at me. I can't help it; it makes my hand shake more when people watch me. I'll just tell them I'm full and then it will be OK, but that taste of drink was real good and the cookie is half dry. No, I don't want to do anything. Everyone is staring.

Good, there's Mom. I can leave. I'm not sure about this and the hateful woman is my teacher Mrs. Gamble and she is old. Maybe I can stay away from the mean girl and the other ones will forget.

I've been in school a couple of weeks now. I HATE SCHOOL!!!!! Mrs. Gamble is mean to me. Mom taught me how to read some and I know my ABC's and my numbers. I knew them before I came to school.

I am in the Redbird reading group and it is the one with the hardest books. That mean girl still makes fun of me and I told Mrs. Gamble, but she told me not to tattle and sit down.

The mean girl, her name is Marie, and she is not in any of my groups and I'm glad!! The girl that has the same name as me is in all my groups and we are best friends. She is real smart and her work always looks so neat. We are learning to write our ABC's the way you are supposed to. I try my best but my A's and H's look awful. I'm trying to hold my pencil tight so it can't shake, but my A's always look squiggly. Mrs. Gamble told me if I didn't quit daydreaming and get my work done faster she is going to change my group. I DO NOT daydream.

I'm trying to go as fast as I can, but if I rush my letters all are squiggly. Mrs. Gamble is standing right behind me. She takes my hand and guides it, and, hey, my letters are pretty. When she leaves, they squiggle again.

I know how I can stay in Jan's writing group. I ask her if she wants me to take her paper to the desk. She said OK. I stop to get a drink and at a worktable I make two lines on her last name initial and it looks like my name. Now I take the eraser and erase the two lines off my paper. It worked! I switched our papers! When I lay the papers on Mrs. Gamble's desk, I put mine on top. She tells me, "Much better. See how neat you can be when you really try."

It's time to go home. I go to my room and just lie on my bed and cry. I just remembered that taking someone else's work is cheating. That is one of the worst things you can do. God doesn't like it! Will He be mad at me, too? What am I going to do?

I don't need to worry. When I get to school the next day, Mrs. Gamble takes my arm and tells Jan to be in charge and everybody study their spelling words. She is really mad 'cause she is hurting my arm. OH NO, the principal's office! I am in trouble. Mrs. Gamble could tell where I had erased part of my last initial. She tells the principal that I am bright but all I do is daydream and then slop through my work to hurry and get it done. The principal calls my mother.

I have to sit there 'til she gets there. The principal tells me to sit still and quit playing with my hands. I'm not playing with my hands, I'm SCARED. My mother comes in and her eyes are red. I made her cry. I CHEATED. Now God is mad at me, too, if my mom is. My mother explains that my father has tremors and I do, too. The principal asks Mom how much my father drinks and why would I have them.

Oh, the principal is in trouble. Mom is mad. She tells me to go wait in the hall, but I want to stay. Mom never gets mad, but when she does, even Daddy sits there and doesn't say a word. I'm in the hall and I can hear my mother talking. She is using her mad voice; she doesn't yell, but it is a different kind of voice. I don't hear the principal. After a little bit, Mrs. Gamble comes to the office and I can hear Mom tell her "And I would like a few words with you, too." It's pretty good to hear Mom telling Mrs. Gamble that she has a few things to tell her. Boy, is she going to get it!

Mom comes out of the office and gives me a hug. She'll see me after school and we will talk about it. Boy, am I going to get it! If Mrs. Gamble and the principal call me in now, I'll get a paddling, I know. Mrs. Gamble is still mad. She must be—her face is red. She is really looking at me mad. She tells me that I will do my work as much as I can and to take the part I don't get done home and finish it. It better look neater than it has been. After that she really doesn't like me. She makes me be last in line all the time and I can't go to the bathroom. When I ask, I have to wait. The work that I don't get finished I take home and have to do as soon as I get there. My answers are always right, but

Mrs. Gamble always writes, "Try to be neater on your papers." I HATE SCHOOL.

The other kids find out and make fun of me at recess. Jan and two other girls play with me. I just don't like being me. What is wrong with me?

I don't give up easy and find out that if I can make the teacher laugh, it's a lot easier. I do have some bad times, really bad, and I cry a lot, but I learn to laugh a lot. I figure out that if I do my work at home where no one is staring at me, I can do better. So I get the assignments from my teachers and do as much as I can the day before class. I get along with the other students by making fun of myself before they can. The ones I go to school with all my life don't pay any attention to my tremors for the most part.

The only time I really want to die is when I have to give a book report or stand in front of the class. I do my best, shaking all over. The ones that I look and see smiling I know are going to tease me but not mean. There are a lot that look at me like they feel so sorry for me. I know those will never have anything to do with me and that hurts. What hurts the worst are the ones who just look disgusted like I'm a freak, and those are the ones that usually call me a freak or shaky lady. Just pick a hateful name and I get called it one time or another. They sometimes stand in a group and laugh when I walk by. That really hurts.

I never eat lunch at school. That is something I

never figured out how to do and not embarrass myself. I get mad, too, but my father said the best way to show someone I'm normal is to make better grades than they do, and as a rule I do. I manage to stay on the A-B honor roll. I think this is as much through anger as brains—I just work harder. One thing that Essential Tremor has given me that is very precious to me is the fact that I love people for who they are, not what they have or who their parents are.

Years Later

I had one heck of a time in college. If I had a lecture class, I took a tape recorder before anyone ever started taking them. I just couldn't take notes fast enough. Then I could go back to the dorm and listen to it again without the frenzy of trying to take notes and correct anything I got wrong. Plus it turned out to be an advantage because I retained more of the lecture than the other students who just went in, did their thing, and left.

I'm no genius, but I kept a decent grade point average for two reasons. First, I was determined to be a liberated female, support myself and never get married, like Mary Tyler Moore. Secondly, and most important, if my average dropped below what my father told me I had to keep, I knew the money stopped—no questions asked. I made it through school pretty well, had some fun. I got my heart broken a couple times; broke a few hearts, too. I had to work harder than most and I played just as hard as any, too. I graduated in the top half of my class.

I was out in the real world and got a standard navy blue interview suit and hit the job market. I had a hard time in the beginning because I was judged by my tremor before I opened my mouth. I thought about this and decided to try taking away any impression before it was made. I went into an interview, shook hands, and then informed the HR director that I had Essential Tremor, that it did not affect my work, and had been an asset to me in the past on judging personalities by their reaction. That worked like a charm. I was employed on the second interview. Plus I appeared to be very professional and spunky. I know, I hate that word but when your 5' 2" and weigh 104 tops, "spunky" fits.

My career was off and so was my marriage to a person who had been a friend for years but had never thought of dating. Don't know what happened, but we got married on February 29th. I never do things like other people; after all, I'm different. I have two grown children who are successful in their own right. Between you and me, I wondered if they would be in bread lines sometimes. I also have six grandchildren: Five are with us and one is with God.

Over the years my tremors have progressed and I had to leave the field I loved. I was asked not to leave by the president of the company, but I felt I wasn't doing as good a job as should be done, and it was due to my tremors, but it beats a life insurance payoff.

I have worked in other less-demanding jobs in the past 10 years, wanting to stay in the workforce, but my tremors became so bad that even with medication no one could read my name when I wrote it. I am in the process of filing for disability; I also have some other medical problems.

I have told my story for a few reasons. The most important reason is to bring awareness to the teaching profession and to the public schools that children with ET are just as smart or even smarter because ET makes you think creatively. Children with ET have some special needs. Teachers and administrators must be educated that ET is the most common movement disorder in the world. How can tens of millions of known cases, and probably at least double undiagnosed cases, be so obscure to so many people? I plan on making sure every school system is knowledgeable on this disorder. I have the future of at least one of my grandchildren at stake, and how many other children do I owe this to? The answer is millions.

Spilled Soup

By Jean Moore

When I was a young adult I can remember noticing

that my mother had a problem signing her name. Sometimes her hand would shake uncontrollably, and she just excused it by saying she must be nervous. I know now that this was her manifestation of Essential Tremor. As far as I know this was her only visible symptom. She was one of the lucky ones. And it was through her genes that Essential Tremor was passed on to me.

My symptoms came on gradually beginning about the age of 40. Little things at first: a slight shaking of the hand when putting a fork to my mouth; trouble holding a cup of coffee steady; and my beautiful handwriting began to change.

Over the next few years these symptoms became more pronounced. When eating, I had to really concentrate to hold my fork steady. Eating soup was nearly impossible. I would have to put my mouth down very close to the bowl to keep from spilling. Drinking any kind of beverage had to be done two-handed. A glass of water or a cup of coffee in one hand could rarely reach my mouth without splashing everywhere. My hand would shake uncontrollably and could only be steadied by the touch of my other hand. Worst of all, at times my handwriting was almost illegible because my hand shook so badly. But this was not consistent. There were times when I could write perfectly fine. But if I was in a hurry, or stressed, or trying to be especially neat—forget it. My hand would not only shake, it would occasionally have spasms.

Despite all of these increased symptoms, I managed to hide my Essential Tremor from my friends and coworkers. I became a master of illusion. When dining out at a restaurant, I would manage to quickly take a bite of food when no one was watching. Ordering soup was out of the question. Holding a beverage with two hands didn't seem such an unusual thing to do, so it didn't raise any eyebrows. On the job, I would type absolutely everything I could. My ET had no effect on my typing. If I did have to actually write something, I would resort to block print if I could, or hold my hand with my other when nobody was looking.

It had taken about 10 years for my symptoms to develop to this point. I just adjusted my life and learned to live with them. It never occurred to me to talk to a doctor about them. Well, I shouldn't say that. It occurred to me, but I didn't want to. The truth is I was scared to talk to a doctor. I was scared that he was going to tell me that I had some dreadful disease like Parkinson's and I was doomed to a life of convulsive shaking all over my body and that what I was experiencing was just the beginning. The fact is that I was scared to death and getting more scared every day.

About a year later I was browsing a copy of a magazine in the employee lounge. I happened to come upon an article that would change my life forever. The article was written by a woman who had a condition called Essential Tremor. As I read on I noticed a lot of similarities between her symptoms and mine. Not just similarities—some of them were identical to mine! And then she went on to say that there were a lot of people who had this condition. And there was treatment for it and it could get better! I was beginning to feel hope. She gave a Web site that was devoted to this "Essential Tremor" and I couldn't wait to get on the Internet.

I went to www.essentialtremor.org and a wealth of information opened up to me. Somehow I just knew that this is what had been the cause of all my dreadful shaking all these years—and it even had a name! It was not Parkinson's disease or even related to it. It was a genetic disorder that I must have inherited from a parent. Only then the memories of my mother's shaky hand came flooding back to me. Of course—she had it, too! I read on and found that Essential Tremor manifests itself differently in every victim. I should count my blessings—I could have it a whole lot worse. The Web site went on to discuss the various drugs that are used to treat ET with considerable success. I printed out several pages and tucked them away.

I had never consulted my doctor about my shaking. I never liked going to the doctor and only went when I was sick enough to need antibiotics. Even though I now knew what I had and that there was treatment for it, I still did not seek help. It was a couple of years later, when my shaky hand finally started affecting my work, that I decided it was time to do something about it.

I worked in a payroll office and needed to post hours. My hand would shake so badly that I could no longer read my own numbers. It was time. I went to my doctor and told him I had a tremor in my hand when I tried to write. He immediately referred me to a neurologist who I saw the next week. After a few simple tests, he confirmed my suspicions. He gave me some information printed directly from the ET Web site and I told him that I already had it all. He seemed pleased that I had done my homework.

Instead of treating me with the conventional drugs, he gave me some samples for a relatively new drug that was generally used for treating epilepsy called Topamax. I started on a very small dose and gradually increased it over time. My symptoms improved as the doses increased. I have been on Topamax for about four years and there is a remarkable decrease in my shaking.

The tremor is by no means totally gone. I would have to say there is about a 50 percent improvement. In times of stress or if I am rushed, my handwriting is still quite shaky. I still need to hold a cup of coffee with two hands, but the shaking is definitely better. And I can now manage to get a forkful of food to my mouth without spilling. I don't think my doctor is through increasing my dosage of medication, so I'm hopeful there may be more improvement in the future.

I have three grown daughters. Of course, they are aware of my struggle with Essential Tremor. Unfortunately, one or all of them may expect to fall victim to my same fate. But at least they will know what it is when the first symptoms appear. At least they will not need to live in fear as I did. I pray that the toss of the genetic dice has been lucky for them, but if it hasn't, at least they will be armed with the knowledge to make their lives manageable.

Spreading the Word

Life-altering events are often difficult to pinpoint in time. Most of us recognize them only with 20/20 hindsight. Unlike most of us, John Cox remembers exactly when one happened for him.

It was late evening on June 13, 2003. That afternoon John's doctor had told him a recent MRI was normal and that there was nothing wrong with him. It was not the first test John had ever had trying to figure out what made his head shake; over the past 27 years he had been tested for nearly everything. And this was not the first doctor to tell him there was nothing wrong.

That evening, John typed "head tremors" into a search engine and waited. The first listing was the International Essential Tremor Foundation (IETF)

Web site. He clicked on it. A life-altering event had begun. John remembers it clearly.

"I started going through the site and I thought, "Oh, my gosh, this is what I have!" His shouts of joy woke Marguerite, his wife.

The next day John called his doctor. Looking at the information John had gotten from the Web site and considering that John's grandmother and all of his cousins had what was called "the shakes," the doctor agreed that Essential Tremor was a possibility.

Soon after, John joined the IETF and read an article about Topamax in an issue of *Tremor Talk* [Ed note: The official IETF newsletter]. He called his doctor again, this time for a prescription.

"It was like getting a new life!" John remembers. "Before, one barber wouldn't cut my hair because I couldn't hold my head still, and a dentist couldn't work on my teeth. People stared and would ask why I was shaking in the middle of summer."

Medication changed all that, eliminating what John estimates to be at least 70 percent of his head tremor. In addition, his health and appearance are improved and his doctor is happy.

Health is only part of it, John says. Knowing he's not alone is as important. "I'm sorry other people have ET, but I'm so glad to know I'm not the only person who has this condition. John wishes he had known in middle school what he learned that June. "I didn't know what I had, but I let it get the best of me," he says.

An accomplished singer, John toured with God-spell and Jesus Christ Superstar. "My understudy is on Broadway today. I should have been there." Instead, he aimed his artistic talent in another direction and became a chef. Attaining a certain amount of recognition in a time of "celebrity chefs," as John describes it, meant TV appearances. "My head shake was so bad, I couldn't do TV when they asked me."

After 18 years as a chef, John switched careers to become something he always wanted to be: an over-the-road truck driver. Now he's spreading the word about Essential Tremor across the miles every week.

Asked what advice he would give to others who have ET, John's answer is quick: "Tremor is what you have; it's not who you are. Don't worry about what other people say or do. I know that's difficult when people are pointing and staring at you, but you just have to keep going. You just have to be yourself and keep going."

John and Marguerite have two sons: Stephen, 20, and Anthony, 10. Both are artists and both have ET. "I'm trying to teach them not to freak out about it," John says. "I'm trying to teach them what I wish I would have known."

No, It's Because You're Old

By Kathy Dudek

My seventh grade English teacher, Mr. Post, was the first person to make an issue of my tremor. Both my father and his father lived with the tremor, but Mr. Post's concern gave ET a name for my family. Because of his suggestion, I had my first visit to a neurologist who told my family I had Essential Familiar Benign Tremor.

Years later when I finished high school, I went to school to receive certification as a dental assistant. The administration tried to discourage me from continuing the program because of my tremor. I finished anyway. However, later while working as a dental assistant, the dentist felt that my tremor was affecting my work more and more so I lost my job. I went to the local job rehabilitation office in the hopes they would guide me by choosing a new direction to go for future employment. I knew being a dental assistant was in my past.

There were other ET-related events in my life, but the one that most affected me was in September of '88. I had decided to return to college. A friend, knowing of my tremor, told me of an office on campus that provided services for another friend with a disability. She was sure I would be eligible to have a note-taker for my classes. As it turned out, I was. I couldn't hold back the tears. Finally, at the age of 35, someone was offering me help with my tremor.

I couldn't have made it through college without the note-takers I had in each of my undergrad classes.

Due to my handicap, I was allowed to do my comprehensive exams on a computer, with additional time. I failed my certification exam three times—filling in the little bubbles took more time for me. After explaining the problem, I was given permission for an extension on my exam time. Finally, I passed!

When I was in my 20s, the neurologist told me in time I would learn to adapt to my tremor. In ways I have, but some things are still hard—like the occasional cashier who impatiently taps her fingers or begins to ring up the next purchase before I've finished writing my check—that frustrates me. I avoid wine because of the type of glasses the wine is served in. I avoid handwriting and instead type everything possible. I use the fatter pens with the rubber grip and I use a credit card, when possible, to avoid having to write out a check.

As a speech-language pathologist working with three-, four-, and five-year-olds, my tremor is not much of an issue. Recently I began taking asthma medication, which made my tremor worse. One of my students asked me why my hands were shaking. I told him my hands shake a little all the time, but because I had been sick and was taking new medicine the shaking is worse. He responded with, "No, it's because you're old." Out of the mouths of babes… I'm 51, so I had a good laugh that day.

From Peanut Race to ET Activism

Lesa Amsden could never win the peanut race in elementary school. She was about six years old, and the race was her first sign of Essential Tremor. Her diagnosis was still years away. "We had to put a peanut in a spoon and walk to the other side of the room without dropping the peanut. The first person to do that won. I could never hold the peanut on the spoon," Lesa remembers.

Over the next 12 years, Lesa's hand tremors were joined by arm and head tremor. Handwriting, always difficult for her, became even more difficult in high school. Eating was a challenge. She stopped eating in front of everyone, including her family and friends. "I skipped lunch at school," Lesa says. "Essential Tremor is socially embarrassing." She isolated herself.

When Lesa was 15, her family doctor told her the shaking, which worsened with stress, was nerves. "I believed I was just a very nervous individual until I was 18," she says. Lesa remembers vividly the day she stopped believing that. She was driving, and remembers the exact place on the road, when she decided she didn't have a bad case of nerves. "I remember thinking that couldn't be true because other people had the same amount of stress I did and they weren't shaking." Suddenly, Lesa had a mission. She would find a doctor who could tell her what she had.

The mission was short. "The first doctor I went

to told me to touch my nose and touch her hand. I did, and she told me I had Essential Tremor. I have never felt as good as I did that day. Just to hear that I had something that had a name—that it wasn't just my nerves."

Following the diagnosis, Lesa went to a neurologist who prescribed medication. When the medications stopped helping, Lesa went to a neurosurgeon. At 21, Lesa had deep-brain stimulation (DBS) surgery. "It changed my entire life!" she exclaims. DBS removed Lesa's head tremor and greatly reduced tremor in her hands and arms. She eats in public, writes, cooks, and puts on makeup. She's happy. "Actually, I sometimes take the wonderful results for granted. I can't even imagine how I lived like I did for so long."

Finding the IETF was another milestone in Lesa's life. "It was great. I finally knew I wasn't alone," she remembers. Now 26, working full-time, and studying business at Colorado Technical University in Sioux Falls, S.D., Lesa has another mission. She's a one-person dynamo when it comes to educating everyone within hearing distance about ET.

"The more people know about Essential Tremor, the more they will accept it," Lesa says. "I talk about it as much as I can to everybody I know."

A presentation she made as part of a college course has become a regular aspect of the class, even though she's no longer in it. The professor, who had never heard of ET, has her return to speak to other students. Lesa and her neurologist talk about ET and DBS to about 200 medical students at the local hospital every year. She also discussed DBS and ET on a local television news program.

In the fall of 2003, Lesa started an IETF support group. New members continue to arrive at each meeting, bringing total membership to about a dozen. Two people in the group have had DBS.

Lesa's mission is a long-term one. "We have to let people know about ET—what it is exactly and how it affects our lives. The more people know about it, the better off we all will be, especially children. I don't want anyone to suffer the way I did."

Consumed by Tremor

By Shari Finsilver

Why me? What's wrong with me? Why can't I be like everyone else? There probably isn't anyone who doesn't ask these questions when they discover that they have something wrong with them. My first inclination that something was different was when I was 11. In elementary school art class, I could never draw a straight line or a circle that wasn't a bit squiggly. I knew that the other kids could. I just figured that the creative, artistic genes didn't bother to come my way and this was the result.

I didn't pay much attention to this artistic weirdness until I was 12 or 13. Then tremors really began to invade my body and control my actions. No longer could I bring a spoon of soup to my mouth without having the soup spill. My beautiful handwriting appeared to change. I couldn't write in a flowing script or even hold the pen in my hand and let it glide across the paper.

It would have been easy and natural to tell my parents that something strange was happening to me. But for some reason, I chose not to share this information with them—or anyone. I just kept it to myself, suffering silently.

At my graduation from elementary school, families were seated in the school auditorium. Each of the graduates entered the auditorium from the two rear entrances, walking in a processional. Standing in line, I was excited to participate in my first school graduation. I was nervous, probably from just being in front of a large crowd. But I had no idea how this nervousness would soon affect me. Not only were my hands shaking, but as I began to walk into the auditorium, my head began trembling. Whoa! What was this!?! I became self-conscious, assuming everyone was watching me, noticing my head shaking. Soon everyone would be thinking, "What's the matter with that girl?" So I put my head down, down as far as I could to try and stop this insane shaking. When I sat in my seat, it became more obvious. While walking down the aisle, I could make different movements to try and control my head. But when seated, this became a real challenge. I was fidgeting and holding my head and neck very tightly, trying to quiet it. I would cock my head to one side, then hold my head back—all very awkward, exaggerated positions—all the while thinking that everyone was staring at me. It was all I could do to get through the graduation exercise.

My body no longer cooperated or acted "normally." I now had to think about every action I took. I had to constantly figure out strategies. While other "normal" people were probably focusing on their day or the activity that they were participating in, I was continuously dreaming up ways to divert people's attention so they wouldn't see my shaking hands. I would devise different methods of doing tasks that involved my hands. Or I lied or came up with deceptions and different tricks so they didn't know I couldn't participate in activities because of my trembling hands. All the while, the truth would have been easier and would have freed up my mind, eased my tension, and relaxed my body. Deception, disguise, and lying were my tools.

Everyone knows that kids just want to fit in. The last thing we want is to be different, especially if we have no choice. Well, I had to work very hard to hide my problem. Every day was a challenge. How do I grab papers from the boy sitting in front of me as they're being passed around the room and then pass them on to the next person behind me? My hands shook so badly that it wasn't easy to hide. Everyday tasks were a huge challenge for me: writing, carrying a lunch tray, putting on makeup.

Chemistry and physics classes were really tough. Can you imagine being in a classroom doing experiments, pouring chemicals from a container in one hand into a beaker being held by the other hand? The only way I knew that I could get through those two classes was to simply not sign up for them. Today that would be impossible. You cannot go to college without high school chemistry and physics. But it wasn't a problem in the 1960s.

Another horrific challenge was what to do when I was called upon to write my answers to a math problem on the blackboard. I still shudder when I think of this! I was a very good student, very competitive, a high achiever. In order not to suffer the humiliation of not being able to scratch out anything legible on the board, I simply told the teacher I didn't know the answer.

Worse yet was Latin class. When asked to be prepared the next day to write that night's translation assignment on the board, I panicked. I did not know how to handle this situation. The only remedy I had was to fake illness and stay home from school. I missed an entire day of school because I couldn't bear the thought of being in front of the class for a couple of minutes or, banish the thought, of actually being truthful with my teacher. I couldn't even tell my parents.

Eating out with friends was tricky. I could only eat sandwiches because they didn't require me to bring a fork up to my mouth. I would hold the sandwich with both hands, place both elbows on the table (sorry, Emily Post), and bring the sandwich to my mouth. I drank with straws and never actually held the glass. I bent over the glass and sipped from the straw. No one ever noticed.

Unfortunately, neither did my parents or sister. We ate dinner together almost every night and somehow I deceived them for years. But the moment of truth had to come sometime and it did one night in 1969 when I was 19 years old. I was sitting across a very long table from my mother, during a large family holiday meal. Somehow my hand just lost control and the fork flew from it. I can still remember the look on my mother's face—shock, horror, and fear. She immediately thought I had Parkinson's disease, which was the natural reaction then and, unfortunately, still today.

She took me to a neurologist, who diagnosed me with Benign Familial Tremor. This is how they referred to Essential Tremor, also called Heredity Essential Tremor. I was fortunate to be diagnosed with

ET by the first doctor I saw. By talking to people who have ET, I have learned that the majority go to several doctors before being properly diagnosed, while many never receive an accurate diagnosis.

The doctor prescribed Librium, a tranquilizer. I took it for awhile, but it didn't help my tremor at all, so I stopped. I did not want to take ineffective medication.

Living with ET has given me the opportunity to become quite an expert on it. I have discovered what triggers make the tremors worse. Adrenaline is the real enemy. Just a shot from being startled, excited, exercising, dancing, or being frightened whip the usual shaking into a frenzy. Or just being cold, tired, or hungry. I couldn't win. For me, the morning was worse, especially right after waking. I became a bit steadier and controlled as the day wore on.

My worst nightmares were always of my wedding and taking care of children. I could not imagine being able to walk down the aisle without my hands, head, and body shaking uncontrollably. And, worse yet, I was horrified to think that I might not be able to hold and feed my babies. But my worst fear was that in an emergency, I wouldn't be steady enough to help my children.

College years are known as a period of great self-discovery. For me, I found how best to calm the shaking. Alcohol! I actually never grew fond of drinking, but did find out by accident that alcohol quiets the tremors tremendously. So whenever I really needed to, I would have a drink or use Valium to help me get through dinner engagements, meetings, presentations, and parties. After the occasional use of alcohol and tranquilizers for 30 years, I required higher dosages, even for the short window when I would need relief. Unfortunately, the higher dosage would affect me for as much as two days. This was not acceptable.

Fast forward to 1990 when I turned 40. For some reason, probably hormonal, my tremors got much worse. They were really out of control. I was beginning to require two hands to eat using utensils; my arms were now affected; the head tremor, which really only occurred occasionally up to now, was getting worse; my voice was now affected so that it shook when I was speaking publicly or on the telephone; and I could feel a constant tremor internally. If you touched my body when I was nervous, you could feel it vibrating.

I just couldn't take it anymore. Every moment was consumed with thinking about my ET. It was really taking a toll on my family. An ET patient cannot cope without a strong support system and I certainly had that with my husband and two children. They ran interference at any function we attended. If someone was passing a plate of food around the table, their hands would immediately extend across me and grab for it, so I wouldn't have to. If food or drink needed to be served to a guest, they would automatically jump up and do it, so I wouldn't suffer the embarrassment. But I was now becoming more and more reclusive because it was so difficult to eat with people. We are very social people, with a large network of friends and family, and very active in our community. Little by little, I had changed the course of our lives with my ET. Instead of being forthright about it, making people comfortable by just talking about it and allowing everyone to see me as I really was, we just stopped being with people.

The various medications available for ET patients never reduced or controlled my tremors. So I turned to exploring all the options that non-traditional medicine had to offer. Over many years, I tried acupuncture, dietary changes, nutritional supplements, hypnotherapy, chiropractic, Reiki, and different forms of exercise. Although none of these therapies stopped my shaking, I gained something positive from each one and have since incorporated many of them into my daily life.

A miracle did occur for me when my sister sent me a tape of the show "20/20," highlighting a newly approved procedure called deep brain stimulation (DBS) surgery. I eventually had this electrical stimulation system implanted in my brain and abdomen, which controls my tremors during waking hours. This surgery has been a life-altering experience, allowing me to live life free of tremor. Like someone awakened from a lifetime coma, I immediately began doing all the things I had not been able to do for 40 years: write by hand, use a camera, cut with scissors, make change at the cash register, sign checks and credit card receipts, enroll in a public speaking course, dance with men other than my husband and son—all the things most people take for granted.

I also decided to start a support group, sponsored by the International Essential Tremor Foundation, in my local area so that other people with ET would never have to feel alone, embarrassed, and different like I did.

But, best of all, I was able to walk down the aisle at my children's weddings, beaming with love and pride, and cradle my grandchildren in my arms with steady hands.

Someone Who Understands

By Shirley Watts

I started noticing my shaking when I was in the sixth grade. That was my last year of eating in the lunchroom. I went through middle and high school and never ate in the lunchroom with my friends again. I was so paranoid because of my shaking that I just could not make myself eat in front of people.

My parents did not know I wasn't eating at school and continued to give me a check each week for my lunch money. I cashed the check at school and spent the money. In high school I started smoking so that was where I spent my lunch money. I spent the entire lunch period in the bathroom.

It seems I have spent my whole life around my shaking. My parents took me to doctors when I was in the ninth or tenth grade. I was put in the mental part of a hospital in Birmingham, Ala. I guess they thought I had mental problems because I told them I was nervous.

When my daddy taught me to drive I shook all over. Anything I did or do that makes me nervous, I shake worse. When I was sent to the store for something, I panicked so bad I felt like I was going to faint. Do you know why? It is because I wouldn't want them to see my hand shaking when I exchanged money with the cashier. When I did have to do that I used the line, "Oh, I'm just nervous because I have a dentist appointment."

I never felt like all my friends. I had to work everything around my shaking. We once went on a field trip to Ft. Tucker, Ala., a U.S. Army base. The bus dropped us off at the base and everyone got off to eat lunch in the mess hall except guess who? Me. I was so hungry, but you could not have gotten me off the bus.

When I started dating and we drank beer, I discovered something that made me feel calm. We drank on the weekends some but not excessively. When I drank two or three beers I felt like I wasn't scared to do things, like eat in a restaurant and all.

I got married in 1975 to my one true love and we are still together and have two daughters, 24 and 27. I was not diagnosed with ET until the '80s by a neurologist in Montgomery, Ala. His name is Dr. Cox. I really liked him. But do you know that even though he told me I had Essential Tremor, I thought I was the only one who had it? I was put on medication twice a day.

Two years ago I was at the ballpark and this woman began talking to me and I told her about my shaking. Sometimes you just want to talk to someone about it, I guess. The next time I saw her she handed me some material she had gotten off the Internet about ET. I could not get home fast enough to read it.

I realized that what I have, other people do, too, and it really is not just "my nerves." I called the number on the papers she gave me and it was to the International Essential Tremor Foundation (IETF). The IETF sent me information about ET.

My whole life has revolved around my shaking. For years I would not eat in a restaurant. When I finally started doing it, I had to find a spot that I could sit with my back to everyone. Now I try not to think about it so much and my husband and I eat out all the time. I have found that if we go with a group of people I will start worrying that I'm going to be nervous so I wind up being even more shaky.

Finally, I would like to share the times I shake and what shakes. I definitely wouldn't join a gym again. I did once and my first day I was the only one in the gym for about 15 minutes. When I left I could hardly walk to my car, my legs, arms, everything was shaking so badly. I have learned living with ET that there are some things in life you just can't do. When I am really upset, my head shakes and my talking is so bad I feel like a freak. My lips and jaw will shake; I learned that from going to the dentist when I have to hold my mouth open. When I lay my hands down and try to hold my thumbs up, they go crazy.

I don't work outside the home. My husband has his own construction business and we do pretty well so I don't have to work. But I would love to work somewhere like Wal-Mart or a department store just so I could have my own spending money. But I am so paranoid about my shaking that I don't.

We will be having our first grandbaby soon and I am terrified that just holding her for a few minutes my hands will shake. I am also afraid because I know the older I get, the worse my tremors will get. I could not begin to tell you all the times in my life my shaking screwed things up, embarrassed me, or kept me from doing things other people do.

I definitely try not to dwell on it or feel sorry for myself like I used to do. If I do, I get depressed. My big fear is that it will turn into Parkinson's one day (Author note: While someone with ET may also develop Parkinson's disease, ET cannot turn into Parkinson's disease). If it does, I don't want to live like that. I just thank God I'm still here and can do all the things I can do and I am so glad I know about the IETF now. I don't feel so alone as I had my whole life. Thanks for reading this. That's all I wanted, someone to read this who truly understands.

Man, You've Got the Shakes Bad

By Steven Reigns

Had I been bookish-looking or had I spent my social time differently, maybe it would have been more socially awkward to shake continually. At 16, I abandoned the library and all academic aspirations to become a partier. With the help of Shawn King's Missouri driver's license, my real age knew no bounds—thanks to his birth five years before me. I soon found the crowd my mother warned me about and courted them until I was accepted. After that, my adolescent years were spent in a blur of bars, clubs, raves, after-hour parties, and sneaking into concerts.

I'm not sure when my shaking started. My parents were too concerned with how I wasn't fulfilling their parental athletic dreams to focus on the steadiness of my hands. I always had bad handwriting, so gauging writing samples doesn't help either. By 16, my shaking was considerably more noticeable. I lived with it for so long that it didn't occur to me that shaking was abnormal. It was common to me.

Soon I was invited to the hottest clubs and hung out with the hottest crowd. It was a seedy scene of bar stars and drug users. Befriending such a group of delinquents, I didn't expect my shaking to even be noticed. And thankfully, it hardly ever was. But it was in the early morning, after an all-night party that a drunken guy commented to me, "Man, you've got the shakes bad. Coming down is a bitch."

He wasn't referring to medication given by doctors, he was referring to the type of drugs that would crowd bathroom stalls with everyone trying to get some of the action. This wasn't someone asking if I was nervous or had Parkinson's, as a women in the grocery store asked me one day. His assumption made me feel included in the social group and even gave me the edge of being rebellious and daring. He thought I was a hardcore drug user. Such an extreme user that I'd boldly stay at this early morning party with the "detox shakes." This was the first time my tremors were thought to be drug induced and the association was welcomed. The negative social stigma of drug abuse seemed far less important to me than a young person with an unattractive hand tremor problem.

My life settled down when I moved and attended college. By then I was more interested in academics than partying. It was during this shift of environment and social crowd that more people commented on my shaking. I became increasingly self-conscious. In class, I'd place my hands on my lap below the desk, take notes sparingly, and always type out reports.

I'd like to have drawn upon a pinnacle moment that I sought help, but there wasn't one. I may have been tired of not having an excuse when people asked why I was shaking. When questioned sufficiently about my tremors, I'd admit that I didn't know why I shook and that I had always been that way. This answer never satisfied the questioner and always made the painful reality clear to me: I had no understanding of my body or why my hands shook.

I had an awful relationship with my parents and knew they wouldn't be a resource for information. I went to my physician who told me that "everyone shakes" and that my tremors were just "more pronounced than most people." This appeased me for three years until they got significantly worse. I went to a female neurologist I found in the Yellow Pages.

The neurologist sat behind her desk and told me

that I'd shake for the rest of my life. She said that the shaking might even move up to my neck and head. When I asked if there was any treatment to stop it, she replied, "Get used to it. If you think having money could help you, look at Katharine Hepburn. If she could have fixed it, don't you think she would have?" She told me there was medicine to temper the tremors but one of its major side effects was loss of sexual function. I didn't want to give up my favorite hobby. Not the type of medicine a sexually active, single male in college wants to start using.

I would have preferred being given my diagnosis by someone a bit kinder. But stating that now sounds like the equivalent of someone talking about their ex: "It wasn't that he broke up with me, it was the way he did it."

Choosing to be proactive about answers to my tremors was the first step in becoming more comfortable with my condition. I began researching and reading about my diagnosis with more voraciousness than I had in my earlier party life. I read everything I could on the subject. I discovered the International Essential Tremor Foundation and attended a support group. I was warmly welcomed, but I was the youngest in the room by at least 20 years.

Stories were swapped of misdiagnoses, unneeded surgeries, and inappropriate medication. After hearing the horrors of people treated by the medical establishment years before my birth, I didn't feel a need to talk about my cold doctor and her harsh Hepburn comparison. I hasten to compare emotional states and experiences, but it seemed as if my encounter paled in comparison to the recounts of stories past.

The people before me were those who fought for adequate treatment and wrote letters demanding more research. I felt in good company and remained silent the entire time I was there. A few meetings later, during the sharing part, I asked a question to the males: "Have you experienced sexual side effects from any of the medications?" The small minority of males in the group stared at their shoes, avoiding my question. The lack of a response was answer enough. It also reminded me of the generational difference between us. Had the side effect been dry mouth or diarrhea, the information would have been gladly shared. Since it pertained to sex, the desire to share information did not supersede their generational belief that such talk is embarrassing. It was clear I wasn't in a group of my peers and didn't return.

I still get asked if my tremors are drug detoxification induced. I'm older now and see questions as opportunities to educate. I don't feel a need for excuses, evasiveness, or artificial reasons. What I have is Essential Tremor and that is my reality.

The Unsinkable

By Millie Hess

I have had ET for 16 years. Before that I had beautiful penmanship. When the tremor started, I knew it was not drinking that was making this happen to me. Then I remembered my father shook when he was in his senior years and thought, "Oh nuts, this can't happen to me!"

Well, because of this I am now retired and participate in a singing competition with the Sweet Adelines (singing doesn't put a vibrato in my voice) and volunteer at a food pantry, where we give food to the homeless, unemployed, and low-income. Once a week I volunteer in a hospital, giving directions to about 40 people an hour who don't know where they should go.

Playing dominoes weekly is still possible even though my tremor hangs around. My friends understand. I am part of a boating club where I have helped assemble a cardboard boat that we race in the ocean. I have been in the competition twice and what a great sound to hear "Come on, Millie" as I round the last buoy! My tremor doesn't bother me then. It's running from the flags to the boat where these cute young gals beat me!

I hope I don't see the day my children and grandchildren get Essential Tremor. But only God knows that. I have been in three clinical trials for ET. If there are more chances for me to help in trials in the future, I will!

At 74, I can still dance, but being a widow I prefer line dancing—it's a kick! My plan for the near future is to join a writing class to write down some of my adventures for my grandchildren.

I AM THE UNSINKABLE MILLIE HESS!

Chapter 4
Ways to Cope with Essential Tremor

Essential Tremor (ET) is a life-altering condition that turns simple, everyday acts of living into tests of ingenuity and perseverance. Writing a letter, getting dressed, eating, applying makeup, and handling tools take on a different perspective for people who have ET.

The stress and embarrassment of social situations—eating in public, conducting business meetings, attending wedding receptions—can lead to self-imposed isolation. People who have ET may feel powerless about controlling tremor, which can cause more stress. They may feel depressed or sad because they don't feel they have the tools to deal with the condition. People who have ET may have difficulty with basic daily activities. For example, writing, dressing, cutting food, handling utensils, and eating certain foods. As a result of ET, people may restrict their activities to those that involve only people very close to them. They don't go out to dinner because someone might stare or because they might spill. Some have even passed up work promotions because the new responsibilities would include conducting business meetings and luncheons. Although the information here won't solve your difficulties, it will provide ideas that will not only help you cope, but also may help trigger coping ideas of your own. These tips should not replace your current medical therapy, but they may enhance the treatment process. Be sure to discuss your difficulties with your physician or other healthcare professional to help develop a well-rounded treatment plan that is right for you.

Tips from IETF Members

What better source of ideas for living with ET than people who have the condition and the people who love them? The following are practical suggestions from IETF members.

Eating and drinking

- If your dominant hand shakes, teach yourself to use the other hand to eat and hold a cup or glass.

- If you have head tremor, hold your chin toward your chest to help steady your head.

- To hold a mug or small glass, put your thumb along the rim and the four other fingers underneath.

- Pick up cups and mugs from the top with all five fingers.

- Use eating utensils that have large handles.

- Use a 1 in.-deep dish that has vertical sides.

- Hold your drinking glass in the palm of your non-dominant hand and steady it with your dominant hand.

- Eat with the utensil pointing toward you with as much twist to your wrist as you can manage.

- When you carry something containing a liquid, twist your arms and wrists for greater stability.

- Use two hands to hold a soup or cereal spoon.

- Use straws and carry them with you. In restaurants, ask the server to put the glass within easy reach so you can use your straw rather than lift the glass. Be careful when you take the first sip of a hot beverage.

- Fill your coffee cup only half full.

- Eat finger food.

- Ask your dentist for a chain with alligator-clip ends to make a bib of your napkin.

- Tell your priest if you cannot hold the tiny Communion cup without spilling. Ask for a larger glass.

- When you order a meat entrée, ask the server to bring your meal to you with the meat already cut.

- When you order soup, ask for a coffee cup as well and pour the soup into the cup so you can drink it.

- Use travel mugs with tight-fitting lids. Carry one with you, keep one in your car, and give one to each of your friends so they'll have them when you visit.

- Buy a plate bumper guard from a medical supply store. The plastic ring clips onto your dinner plate so you have something to push against to get food onto your spoon or fork. Try eating English or European style (inverting the fork in your non-dominant hand).

- Use a rubberized placemat that sticks to the table.

- Use a plate that has sides three-fourths of the way around.

- Use a bib with a Velcro® closure.

- When you eat milk and cereal, press the spoon down hard into the bowl before raising the spoon to your mouth.

- If you can't drink from a straw without crushing it, make a more durable straw from cane. Cut between the joints, clean out the pith, round the ends, and notch one end similar to a pipe stem.

- When eating, extend your arm perpendicular to the table, flex your elbow, and point your hand to the opposite side of your body.

- Avoid caffeine.

- Use a heavy drinking glass.

Writing

- Simplify your writing style. Printing is easier than script; down strokes are easier than up strokes.

- Change your signature so you can sign your name in a couple of strokes.

- Write in small letters—it's easier than writing in large letters.

- Rest your forearm on a table.

- Try using large, weighted pens.

- Hold the pen between your index and middle finger.

- If you're going to the bank, prepare everything (e.g., filling out forms, signing checks) before you leave home.

- Sit at a desk/table and hold a clipboard (or some similar device) at an angle. Balance the clipboard against the edge of the desk and against your legs.

- Sit on the floor/bed/chair with a clipboard (or some similar device) balanced on your crossed legs.

- Use two hands. Hold the pen or pencil between the thumb and forefinger of one hand and hold about three fingers of your other hand against the pen or pencil.

- Use automatic payments and direct deposit to reduce the number of checks you write and deposit slips you fill out. For example, have utility and health insurance bills automatically deducted from your account and have checks (e.g., Social Security) automatically deposited.

- Use a signature stamp for items that require a legible signature.

- Hold your elbows close to your body.

- Write all your checks on the same day.

- If your dominant hand shakes, teach yourself to write with the other hand.

- Try a Pilot Dr. Grip pen or Sanford PhD pen.

- Place paper on a rubberized placemat that sticks to the desk or table. Not only will the paper stay in place, but you'll be able to press harder.

- Use pre-printed, personalized stationery.

- Have friends sign your name in guest books and on group cards.

Using a Computer

- Use a computer whenever you can and position the keyboard comfortably. Use the mouse.

- Anchor your palms against the front of the keyboard and let your fingers do the walking.

- Set your computer to omit double strikes on the keyboard. Adjust the interval for double-clicking the mouse.

- Attach a wrist rest that allows you to slide your hands as you type so you don't have to lift them.

- Use computer software to write checks.

- Wear wrist weights.

- Try a Kensington Turbo Mouse. It may be easier to use than a regular mouse.

- Use a handheld tape recorder to make notes and then transcribe them on your computer.

- Use a large, square mouse.

- Consider an optical mouse that uses a pad instead of a ball.

Performing Daily Tasks

- Use an electric toothbrush.

- Tell the people at your bank that you have ET.

- Use credit and debit cards instead of writing checks.

- Carry pre-printed labels with your name, address, and phone number.

- Use Velcro® rather than buttons.

- Lean against walls to steady yourself.

- When using the toilet, hug the bowl with your calves while you lower and raise your clothing.

- Use two hands. Hold the object between the thumb and forefinger of one hand and hold about three fingers of your other hand against the object. This applies to razors, toothbrushes, hairbrushes, and a number of daily tasks.

- Use an electric razor.

- Put a filled ice-cube tray into a plastic bread bag and put the whole thing in the freezer. When the cubes are ready, release them into the bag. Remove the tray and empty the bag of ice into the pitcher, glass, or ice bucket.

- Use a tray to carry food and drinks to the table.

- Buy an electric kettle—they're easier to control without spilling. Never fill it more than one-third full.

- Use sugar-substitute pills rather than sugar bowls and dispensers.

- Move your microwave onto the kitchen table so you can slide a plate across the table and only lift it a couple of inches to slide it into the microwave.

- When you buy a telephone, look for one with buttons conveniently configured. Phones that have speed dial and redial buttons in front of the numbers may cause you to press the wrong buttons. Phones that have numbers in the handset allow you to brace one hand against the other.

- Use a speakerphone.

- For things like safe-deposit boxes, have your

physician write a note you can permanently attach to your signature card.

Applying Makeup and Putting on Jewelry

- Rest your elbows on the countertop. Put the mascara wand in one hand and use the other hand to steady it while you apply the mascara.

- Rest a finger of your fisted hand on your cheekbone to put on eyebrow pencil.

- If your hand shakes as it gets near your eye when you apply eyeliner, put the pencil at the starting point, rest your hand against your face, and draw the line from there.

- When applying mascara, eyeliner, and lipstick, steady your hand by resting the palm or a little finger on part of your face.

- Rest your elbows on a table and rest your chin on an upended facial tissue box to help put on earrings.

Taking Care of Yourself

- Follow good health habits, including good nutrition and a balanced diet.

- Educate yourself and others about Essential Tremor. People will be more comfortable when you tell them what you have and explain what it is.

- Accept and admit that you have ET and learn to live with it as best you can.

- Remember that ET, even with all its drawbacks, is not life-threatening.

- Overcome the embarrassment of having ET. That alone can ease the stress and tension that make tremor more pronounced.

- Don't feel guilty about having ET, especially about your children inheriting it. You have no control over that.

- Enjoy and appreciate the times you can do things without tremor.

- Consider meditation, massage, or acupuncture.

- Try not to become overtired, nervous, or stressed.

- To read in bed, hold the paper or magazine in the hand with the tremor and put a finger of your other hand about halfway between the elbow and wrist of the hand holding the paper or magazine.

- Turn your head to the side to control head tremor.

- Wear a foam neck collar during stressful times.

- Form a water-based slab gel into a collar. Cool it in the freezer for comfort during the summer.

- Try breathing exercises to help reduce stress.

- Consider medications that may reduce stress.

- Try biofeedback to help decrease stress that can increase tremor. Ask your neurologist to recommend a psychologist who specializes in biofeedback.

- Count slowly to 10 to relax yourself before beginning a task.

- Chew gum to help control head shaking.

- If you are of legal drinking age, consider a small amount of alcohol to quiet head and jaw tremors before a trip to the dentist.

- During dental procedures, stop periodically to massage and rest your jaw. Ask your dentist whether a bite block will help steady your jaw during dental procedures.

- Talk with your dentist about having a person in addition to the dental assistant help with your procedure. The third person can hold your head gently to calm tremor.

Exercising

Be sure to talk with your physician before beginning any exercise program.

- Follow an exercise program. Exercise may release endorphins, which may help calm tremor, and it can increase your energy level. Exercise can be as simple as a 30-minute walk or as intensive as an hour of aerobics.

- Consider lifting weights.

- Consider stretching. It can help keep muscles limber and reduce spasms. It can also improve your sense of balance.

- Twist your forearms and wrists to give greater stability when you play golf. Grip the putter between your thumbs and forefingers, which will twist your forearms inward, then concentrate on your shoulder turn.

- To tee up a golf ball, first place the tee in the ground. Stand up straight. Bend down again and place the ball on the tee. Try a soft rubber golf tee that has a round base and a tubular stem that supports the ball.

For additional information on living with Essential Tremor, visit the International Essential Tremor Foundation Web site at www.essentialtremor.org or call the IETF to request a tremor reading list at 1-888-387-3667.

Printed in the United States
96447LV00006BA/66/A

9 781598 580914